How to finally shed those extra pounds

HOW TO FINALLY SHED THOSE EXTRA POUNDS:

REMEDY FOR LASTING WEIGHT LOSS

BY

DR MANUEL H. GALLAGHER

TABLE OF CONTENT

INTRODUCTION

According to the most recent WHO forecasts, at least one-third of the world's adult population is overweight, and about one-tenth is obese. Furthermore, nearly 40 million children under the age of five are overweight. Being overweight or obese can have major effects for one's health. Carrying excess fat has major health repercussions, including cardiovascular illness (mainly heart disease and stroke), type 2 diabetes, musculoskeletal problems such as osteoarthritis, and several malignancies (endometrial, breast, and colon) (endometrial, breast, and colon). These disorders result in premature death and substantial disability.

What is not well understood is that the danger of health problems begins when a person is only slightly overweight and that the possibility of difficulties grows as a person's weight increases. Many of these disorders cause people and their families to suffer for a long period. Furthermore, the prices of the healthcare system can be expensive.

The good news is that becoming overweight or obese is largely preventable. The key to success is to achieve an energy balance between calories consumed and calories used on the one hand.

To do this, people can limit the number of total fats they consume, switch from saturated to unsaturated fats, consume more fruits and vegetables, legumes, whole grains, and nuts, and consume less sugar. Additionally, individuals can raise their levels of physical activity, engaging in at least 30 minutes of consistent, moderate-intensity activity on most days in order to burn more calories.

Obesity and overweight are more health issues than cosmetic ones.

ADVANCED DEATH

The projected annual death toll from obesity is 300,000. With weight growth, the risk of death increases.

A person's chance of dying rises with even moderate weight gain (10 to 20 pounds for a person of average height), especially for adults aged 30 to 64.

Compared to persons who are at a healthy weight, obese people have a 50–100% increased risk of dying before their time from any cause.

HEART ILLNESS

People who are overweight or obese have a higher incidence of heart illness, including heart attacks, congestive heart failure, sudden cardiac death, angina or chest discomfort, and irregular heart rhythms.

Those who are obese are twice as likely to have a high blood pressure as adults who are at a healthy weight.

Increased triglycerides (blood fat) and lower HDL cholesterol is associated to obesity ("good cholesterol") ("good cholesterol").

CANCER

A increased risk of certain malignancies, such as endometrial (uterine lining cancer), colon, gall bladder, prostate, kidney, and postmenopausal breast cancer, is connected to being overweight or obese.

Compared to women whose weight is stable, those who gain more than 20 pounds between the ages of 18 and middle age have a twofold greater chance of getting postmenopausal breast cancer.

RESULTS OF LOSS OF WEIGHT

In overweight or obese person, weight loss as minor as 5 to 15% of total body weight might lessen the risk factors for several diseases, most notably heart disease.

Blood pressure, blood sugar, and cholesterol levels can all be improved with weight loss.

If a person has a Body Mass Index (BMI) that is higher than the healthy weight range*, weight loss may be beneficial, particularly if that person also has other health risk factors like high blood pressure, high cholesterol, smoking, diabetes, a sedentary lifestyle, and a personal or family history of heart disease.

CHAPTER 1

OVER WANT AND OVER STARVING (WHY YOUR BODY IS ALWAYS HUNGRY)

The hunger hormone is another name for ghrelin. Although the brain, small intestine, and pancreas also create a minor quantity, the stomach produces the majority of it. When the stomach is empty, the production of ghrelin increases, and the blood sugar level begins to decline. This translates to the fact that ghrelin levels in the blood are normally high before meals and begin to fall as the stomach fills up.

Ghrelin production is reduced more by meals high in high-quality fiber and protein than by simple carbs like sugar and honey or by fatty foods. This is one reason why, if you eat foods that are heavy in sugar and fat, you could occasionally ingest more calories than you need. Although the specific mechanism is uncertain, one method that bariatric surgery benefits in weight loss is by generating a decrease in ghrelin levels. This means that the impulses to the brain that produce hunger are also altered, in addition to the amount of food that can fit in the stomach.

Being a foodie is distinct, and being continually enticed to eat something is a whole different feeling. It's conceivable for someone to continually want to try new things or experiment with different cuisines, while another individual may only require food to binge on. People who fall into the latter category frequently still feel hungry hours after finishing their meals. Here are a few reasons why you could always feel as though you could eat a horse if you're one of those people who are perpetually hungry.

You overindulged during supper. Crabs tend to be taken into your body as sugars quite fast when you eat more than is necessary at once. The release of insulin is triggered by a quick spike in blood glucose levels. And as a result, all sugar is processed more quickly by the body, which gives you an overpowering want to eat more carbohydrates. This occurs as a result of increased insulin synthesis, which produces a fast drop in blood sugar. And you can wake up in the middle of the night feeling terribly hungry.

HORMONES

Hormones have a key function in modulating both hunger and metabolism. The thyroid gland performs a critical function in maintaining the body's homeostasis. Your body burns more calories than usual when your thyroid is overactive, which may make you feel more hungry. Graves' disease is a serious disorder that results in the overproduction of thyroid hormone, driving your body into overdrive and generating unpleasant symptoms including increased perspiration, anxiety, and hunger.

PREGNANCY

An further key cause in increased hunger is pregnancy. Although early pregnancy nausea is a typical symptom, early pregnancy appetite is also a common side effect due to the need to ingest more calories. The early indicators of pregnancy for those who don't suffer morning sickness can include hunger and weight gain.

LACK OF SLEEP

Overeating, obesity, and overweight have all been linked to lack of sleep. Lack of sleep might cause your ghrelin levels, which boost appetite, to rise. For many reasons, obtaining decent sleep is vital. This is just another rationale for shutting out at least 7 to 8 hours per night.

MEDICATIONS

Additionally, taking certain drugs may make you feel more hungry than usual. Steroids are medications that are used to treat a number of inflammation-related illnesses. Long-term use can promote weight gain because it makes you feel more hungry. But it may be treated by practicing mindfulness and avoiding from overeating. The appetite can be boosted by various drugs, particularly somc antidepressants. It's vital to be aware of this and actively control it. While addressing your mental health, you don't want to damage your physical health and enhance your risk of obesity.

KEY CONCLUSIONS:

More than only the actual need for food and nutrients can create hunger.

Typically, when we think of hunger, we think of the need for a meal or a snack. Hunger serves as a cue for you to eat to satisfy your body's requirement for food and energy while you are eating primarily for survival. However, there are situations when we don't really need to eat or ingest any calories at all. Read on to know more.

WHY DON'T YOU KEEP EATING?

The primary cue from the body to stop eating is leptin. Fat cells produce leptin for us. Fat cells expand slightly as a result of eating, which causes them to store extra energy. When that occurs, the fat cells generate leptin, which then travels to the hypothalamus in the brain to let you know you've had enough food and is good to stop eating.

IS HAVING A SEVERE HUNGER PANG NORMAL?

It depends, is the response. Your body requires extra energy in the form of calories to retain its present size if you have been exercising more than normal. Similar to this, dieting has been proven to initially boost ghrelin levels, making you feel hungrier. This contributes to the difficulties of keeping a diet. However, your body tends to recalibrate the parameters of what seems normal after a month or so of eating less.

HEDONISTIC DINING

The phrase "hedonic eating," which was first used in 2007, defines what happens when you continue to eat after feeling full. It occurs when eating and drinking are done more for enjoyment than for hydration and nutrition. The desire to feel good as well as the need to cope with negative emotions can both lead to this type of eating.

MOOD-DRIVEN EATING

The urge to avoid and deal with negative feelings like depression, anxiety, and sadness can lead to emotional eating. Emotions have a lot to do with the hypothalamus, the area of the brain that processes signals that cause a person to feel hungry or full. Eating particularly sweet or fatty foods can release hormones that make you feel happier or satisfied, at least momentarily. Reinforcing this response over time can result in obesity and overweight, which are sometimes seen in conjunction with depressive state.

CHAPTER 2

WHY DO YOU CONSUME BAD FOOD?

Junk food is manufactured with a lot of preparation and money. Junk food is also designed with a lot of effort. The objective is to make it affordable and useful. And even though it delivers little to no nutritional benefit, the objective is to keep you going back for more. It usually has high levels of salt, sugar, and fat. They kick off our brains' pleasure regions, giving us a wonderful high and motivating us to consume more. You see, our brains are fairly huge. They need a lot of energy to fulfill their aims. Thus, we have developed to love high-energy foods. Beyond the unusually high calorie content, junk food makers have a ton of ingenious techniques to make their products enticing. Similar to the trickery, We feel the calories have miraculously vanished. Or enhancing flavor till it approaches "sensory specific satiety." It has a flavor that is so powerful that it confuses your brain. And you ultimately cease desiring. Junk food can consequently be incredibly difficult to avoid, despite the fact that consuming it is connected to illnesses like obesity, diabetes, heart disease, and even cancer.

THE DRAWBACKS OF JUNK FOOD AND FAST FOOD

Junk food is defined as food and beverages that are high in calories, fat; sugar, and/or salt but have minimal nutritional value (such as vitamins, minerals, and fiber) (such as vitamins, minerals, and fiber). Fast food, on the other hand, is a category of food that you can order from a restaurant and is designed to be brought to you as quickly as possible. While the majority of fast food is often junk food, some quick foods can be healthful. Salads, sushi, and sandwiches are a few examples of healthful fast food. However, the majority of fast food outlets, like McDonald's or KFC, sell fatty junk food. In Australia, junk food accounts for 41% of a child's daily energy intake and 35% of an average adult's.

Although consuming junk food once in a while won't cause much harm, frequent consumption has been related to an elevated risk of obesity and chronic diseases. Excessive consumption of junk food is a contributing factor in cardiovascular disease, type 2 diabetes, nonalcoholic fatty liver disease, and some malignancies. Additionally, the exact elements in a number of fast foods might have adverse impacts on your body; \s• Junk food heavy in sodium can cause headaches and migraines to become more common. Junk food heavy in carbs can promote outbreaks of acne

• Consuming too much junk food may increase your risk of experiencing depressed.

• The sugar and carbs in junk food might cause tooth cavities that may require treatment from your family dentist.

• Trans fats included in fried foods elevate LDL cholesterol levels.

• The empty carbs in fast food can result in higher blood sugar levels and insulin resistance.

THE SECRET TO A HEALTHFUL DIET | THE CONSEQUENCES OF JUNK FOOD

Your food must be nourishing and varied if you want to lower your risk of acquiring unfavorable health impacts. Small dietary alterations might have a tremendous influence on your health. It's simpler than you would expect, particularly if you adhere to at least six of the eight objectives outlined below.

• Make half of your plate fruits and veggies. The more colorful your dish is, the more probable it is that you will acquire the vitamins, minerals, and fiber your body demands (such as tomatoes, sweet potatoes and broccoli) (such as tomatoes, sweet potatoes and broccoli).

• Make half of the grains you consume whole grain; doing so will help you avoid processed grains that are heavy in empty carbs. Search for whole wheat, brown rice, quinoa, wild rice, bulgur, buckwheat, oatmeal, rolled oats, or other whole grains.

• Change to low-fat (1%) or fat-free milk: The same amount of calcium and other nutrients are present in fat-free and low-fat milk as in whole milk, but less calories and less saturated fat are present.

• Pick a range of foods with lean protein: Meat with a lower fat content, or lean meat, is much preferable to meat with a higher fat content. Choose thinner cuts of beef, chicken, or turkey breast.

• Sodium in food comparison Choose foods with reduced salt content by considering the nutritional information contained on the labels of food packaging. Select canned foods with low sodium, reduced sodium, or no salt added claims on the label.

• Avoid consuming sugary beverages and instead choose for water or unsweetened liquids to dramatically lower your calorie intake. Avoid sodas and energy drinks because they contain a lot of calories and extra sugar. If you want to give your glass of water some extra taste, try adding a piece of lemon, lime, or watermelon.

• Eat some seafood because it's high in protein, minerals, and omega-3 fatty acids. Seafood comprises fish, shellfish, and mollusks (healthy fat) (healthy fat). If you're an adult, try consuming at least eight ounces of seafood each week.

• Limit your consumption of solid fats, which are typically found in processed meat, ice cream, cakes, and pastries. To limit your consumption of solid fats, aim to avoid these.

The eight aims outlined above will help you reduce unhealthy content while supporting your body in acquiring the nutrients it needed. Your physical and mental health will start to considerably improve if you mix a nutritious diet with frequent exercise.

IMPACT ON THE CARDIOVASCULAR AND GASTROINTESTINAL SYSTEMS

The majority of fast food—including beverages and sides—is heavy in carbs and includes little to no fiber.

The carbohydrates in these foods are released into your bloodstream as glucose (sugar) via your digestive system. Your blood sugar rises as a result.

Your pancreas releases insulin in reaction to the surge in glucose. Insulin transports sugar to the cells in your body that require it for energy. Your blood sugar levels return to normal when your body consumes or stores the sugar. This blood sugar process is closely regulated by your body, and as long as you're healthy, your organs can correctly handle these sugar increases.

However, consuming a lot of carbs frequently can cause your blood sugar to increase repeatedly.

These insulin spikes may eventually decrease your body's regular insulin response. You face an increased chance of developing type 2 diabetes, insulin resistance, and weight gain as a result.

FAT AND SUGAR

Sugar is routinely added to fast food dishes. That means excessive calories as well as poor nourishment. The American Heart Association (AHA) advises ingesting no more than 100 to 150 calories per day from added sugar. That translates to around six to nine teaspoons.

The volume of many fast-food beverages is well above 12 ounces. Eight teaspoons of sugar are included in a 12-ounce can of soda. 140 calories, 39 grams of sugar, and nothing else are present in that. Tran's fats are never beneficial or healthful in any level. It can increase your LDL (bad cholesterol), lower your HDL (good cholesterol), and raise your risk for type 2 diabetes and heart disease. Eating meals containing it can also do these things. Restaurants might make the difficulty with calorie counting worse. In one study, respondents who ate at restaurants they deemed to be "healthy" nonetheless significantly underestimated the quantity of calories in their meal.

Sodium

Some people may find that fast food is more appetizing since it contains fat, sugar, and a lot of sodium (salt) (salt). However, water retention can result from diets high in sodium, which is why eating fast food may make you feel bloated, puffy, or swollen.

Additionally harmful to those with blood pressure issues is a diet high in sodium. Sodium can cause your blood pressure to rise and your heart and cardiovascular system to work harder.

Remember that the AHA urges individuals to take no more than 2,300 mg of sodium each day. Half of your days' worth could be discovered in one fast food lunch.

THE RESPIRATORY SYSTEM IS AFFECTED

Weight gain may arise from eating too many calories from fast food. Obesity may develop from this.

Your risk of respiratory disorders, such as asthma and shortness of breath, is raised by fat.

The increased weight can put strain on your heart and lungs, and symptoms could occur even with minimum effort. Walking, climbing stairs, or exercising may cause breathing problems for you.

The likelihood of respiratory issues in children is particularly obvious. According to one study, children who consume fast food at least three times each week had an increased risk of acquiring asthma.

CENTRAL NERVOUS SYSTEM IMPACT

Although fast eating can temporarily ease hunger, the long-term implications are less positive.

People who consume processed foods and fast food are 51% more likely to experience depression than those who abstain or consume them infrequently.

THE REPRODUCTIVE SYSTEM IS AFFECTED

It's probable that the elements in fast food and junk food will damage your fertility.

According to one study, processed food includes phthalates.

Phthalates are substances that can interfere with the actions of hormones in your body. High levels of exposure to these chemicals may cause problems during reproduction, including birth defects.

THE INTEGUMENTARY SYSTEM IS AFFECTED (SKIN, HAIR, NAILS) (SKIN, HAIR, NAILS)

Your diet may affect how your skin looks, but it might not be from the foods you think.

The Mayo Clinic argues that carbohydrates are to blame for acne outbreaks rather than chocolate or greasy foods like pizza. Foods high in carbohydrates because blood sugar surges, and these rapid changes in blood sugar can cause acne.

According to one study, children and teenagers who consume fast food at least three times each week have an increased risk of acquiring eczema. Eczema is a skin ailment that results in itchy, inflammatory patches of skin that are irritated.

THE SKELETAL SYSTEM IS AFFECTED (BONES) (BONES)

Fast fast and processed food's carbs and sugar might make your mouth's acids more acidic. These compounds can destroy tooth enamel. As tooth enamel wears away, bacteria may establish a foothold, leading to cavities.

Obesity can also result in issues with muscle mass and bone density. Obese individuals are more likely to trip and break bones. Maintaining a nutritious diet and engaging in regular exercise are vital for preventing bone loss and strengthening the muscles that support your bones.

THE SOCIAL EFFECTS OF FAST FOOD

Today, it is estimated that more than two thirds of adults in the United States are overweight or obese. Overweight or obese status is also ascribed to more than one-third of kids between the ages of 6 and 19.

Fast food consumption in America appears to be rising at the same time that obesity rates are rising. According to the Obesity Action Coalition (OAC), there are currently twice as many fast food establishments in America as there were in 1970. Additionally, the percentage of obese Americans has more than doubled.

One study revealed that the calorie, fat, and sodium content of fast-food meals essentially haven’t altered over the years, despite efforts to enhance knowledge and make Americans better shoppers.

The rising frequency with which Americans eat out could be hazardous to both the person and the nation's healthcare system.

CHAPTER 3

WAYS TO DETERMINE GENUINE HUNGER

Food supplies us with energy to get through the day, but for many of us, it also brings comfort. But for a variety of reasons, it might be tough to keep ourselves from eating and stop when we're full.

Enjoying your favorite delicacy or settling in for a warm, hearty dinner can bring you a lot of pleasure. But many of us have problems quitting when we're full. It's usually a good idea to satiate hunger, but many of us find it difficult to determine when we've had enough, which can cause us to overeat and occasionally even gain weight.

Do you frequently eat too much? In order to quit eating before you're too full and lose weight, doctors have unveiled a simple self-help tool that you may use to measure how hungry you truly are.

WHAT METHOD CAN YOU USE TO PREVENT BINGE EATING?

All you have to do is envision a scale that evaluates your hunger from zero to ten, with zero representing feeling famished and ten denoting stuffed.

By assessing how hungry you are before you eat, this scale is supposed to lower your odds of indulging in emotional eating, which includes eating for comfort, enjoyment, or boredom, as many individuals do.

Level 4 correlates to mild hunger, and level 6 refers to mild satisfaction. According to dietician Kristina LaRue, the optimal eating range sits between these values.

She followed by noting that if you evaluate your level of hunger as being between 0 and 2, you should be extra cautious of how rapidly you are eating. In this circumstance, you should actively slow down to prevent crossing levels of satisfaction without realizing it. The majority of meat lovers in Britain claim they don't distinguish their fillet steak from their rump.

A healthy habit to acquire is checking your hunger midway through a meal. LaRue clarified: "Don't give up and eat till you pass out if you are full but still have food on your plate. Push your dish away, request a to-go box, freeze leftovers, or compost it as an alternative."

Measure your hunger again after you finish your meal. At the end, you should feel content and satisfied, which shows that you selected the right portion size. Taking a minute to contemplate what you genuinely need is advised if you are tempted to eat despite being full and not physically feeling hungry.

HOW CAN I GET OUT OF THE HABIT OF OVEREATING?

There are strategies to begin breaking the habit of overindulging. Try as much as possible to consider why we kept eating even after we were satisfied.

Eating balanced meals from a variety of food categories and eating every four to six hours is a good approach to do this (depending on your rating on the hunger scale). This allows your body to reestablish a rhythmic eating pattern and allows for normal peaks and dips in satiety. It's difficult to gauge hunger and fullness until your meter has been calibrated.

ARE YOU STILL FAMISHED?

It can be extremely difficult to tell when you're actually hungry and when your mind is just deceiving you. People have long struggled with food temptations, but these days it's even more difficult to resist those hankerings since we can easily order pizza or chicken wings for delivery using smartphone apps. Being cooped up at home also means we have constant access to the food in our refrigerators and pantries.

Although your body is a fairly adept communicator, Janice Hillman, MD, a doctor at

Penn Adolescent and Young Adult Medicine Radnor, says that it can be simple to misinterpret its cues. That's because there might be a thin line separating "that smells really good" from "I need food for energy."

It becomes even harder to distinguish between hunger and fullness when factors like stress and boredom are present, a crucial skill for maintaining a healthy weight and caring for your body is learning how to distinguish between being truly hungry and succumbing to a common eating trigger. To help you eat healthier, here's how to better understand your body's hunger cues.

Hunger is highly individualized, just like most health-related issues. Two people can eat the same exact meal, leaving one person still hungry and the other completely full.

Depending on whether you worked out at home that morning or spent the entire day binge-watching crime documentaries, your nutritional needs can also change from day to day. The secret is to pay attention to and make an effort to comprehend your body's signals of hunger.

Keeping a food diary is one way to achieve this. You'll be forced to identify your eating habits, both good and bad, by keeping a food diary. You might notice, for instance, that you always reach for a bag of candy to cheer you up in the afternoon or that you always order pizza for movie night.

True hunger cues, such as stomach growling, low energy, shakiness, headaches, and difficulty concentrating, occur when you are truly hungry.

Recognizing when to pay attention to those signals is equally crucial so that you can learn how they feel in the future. Make the following columns in a notebook or on the note app on your phone to construct your food diary: \s• What you consume \s• When do you eat?

• The way you felt and what you did while eating

• Look back over your entries a few days later and "Highlight some of the habits that may be a symptom of mistaking hunger for something else, such as boredom or being around food."

•Make a list of the things that typically "cue" you to eat after that. Common triggers for eating include:

• Feeling stressed, such as following a long day at work or an argument with a friend;

• Seeing something you want to eat on a commercial;

• Opening your refrigerator; relying on routines like brewing your favorite coffee every morning; receiving food from a kind neighbor who baked you cookies; boredom or fatigue.

•Remember to keep account of the times in which you sensed actual hunger cues and reward yourself for paying attention to them.

OBSERVING YOUR HUNGER SIGNS

The difficult part now is to say "no" to overeating. When you have a better understanding of your eating patterns, you can start using this information to plan for situations where food will be involved and to prioritize paying attention to your body.

MAKING PLANS

If you never have to say no to tempting food, saying no is much simpler. This does not entail hastily escaping whenever someone offers you a piece of cake. It entails making advance preparations for eating triggers that you find particularly difficult to avoid.

Do you regularly eat snacks while watching your favorite movies at home, for instance? Choose a healthy snack, such as an apple or some nuts. Or do you find yourself going to the fridge a lot? You can regulate your hunger by sipping water with lemon to motivate you to wait for full meals.

If you can't totally avoid it, make an attempt to prepare with a healthier option. Have a nutritious go-to snack on hand, such as veggies and dip or a handful of almonds, if you usually overeat as a result of stress after work.

Keeping an eye on your physique

Planning for all of your snacks and meals is practically impossible because life is unpredictable. It's up to you to judge if you're genuinely hungry when you meet scenarios when you have to choose a meal alternative you hadn't considered.

Following are a few strategies for assessing your body's degree of hunger:

• Doing a head-to-toe body scan to check your physical state and mood;

• pausing to ask yourself whether you're hungry; attempting to be honest with yourself;

• eating more slowly;

• letting your body tell you when it's full

• Avoiding worrying about food by doing something else

DEVELOPING HEALTHY HABITS

It's vital to be patient with yourself while you shift to a healthy lifestyle since habits take time to build. As you acclimate, practice patience with both your body and yourself.

You'll gradually gain a better understanding of your body day by day. Make sure to acknowledge and reward yourself each time you successfully listen (but not with a cookie) (but not with a cookie).

Remember that healthy eating is all about balance; you have some leeway. If it's your birthday, smile and enjoy your cake. Additionally, if you can be a little flexible, you'll be far more likely to follow the plan the rest of the time. You'll be well on your way to a healthier you whether it takes days or weeks to get used to paying attention to your body's hunger cues.

CHAPTER 4

FORMULATING YOUR MEAL PLAN

A well-thought-out eating strategy is necessary to lose weight in a significant and permanent way. For sustained energy during workouts and daily activities, your body requires the proper ratio of calories and nutrition. The secret to losing fat and keeping it off over time is to keep that balance.

The vitamins and minerals your body requires to maintain energy and build muscle are all included in a convenient and delicious menu in a successful weight-loss diet plan. To create a diet plan for weight loss that is specifically tailored to support your lifestyle, objectives, and habits, follow these steps.

STEP ONE: DON'T USE DIET PLANS THAT COUNT CALORIES

Common diet plans specify a daily calorie target. Dieters are expected to stick to a daily intake range and eat meals that are full of the essential nutrients their bodies require to thrive. But many dieters are already doomed to failure by this fundamental tenet. We advise an entirely different strategy to calorie counting.

Why is counting calories daily the wrong way to think about dietary intake?

Each food has a unique number of calories. It becomes challenging to monitor your intake without tedious tracking unless you eat nearly the same thing every day.

There are several occasions when dieters simply can't maintain a strict daily count without giving up enjoyment of social situations, such as going out with friends or going on vacation.

Many diet plans call for a "cheat day" where the dieter is allowed to eat whatever they want without counting calories in order to avoid temptation. Due to one weekly day of indulgence, it is possible to follow a daily restrictive calorie count and still fail to lose weight.

Calorie counts for the day frequently encourage under eating. Dieters strive to maintain calorie deficits by staying within their limits. Too many calories missed have a negative cumulative effect on weight loss efforts.

We advise you to create a diet plan that addresses your nutritional needs in order to maintain a healthy lifestyle rather than setting yourself a daily calorie limit. This strategy is very beneficial for weight loss because it boosts your energy levels, is less strenuous, and gives you the freedom to indulge in whatever you want as long as you do so in moderation.

Everybody has different nutritional requirements depending on their age, weight, level of activity, and other medical requirements. You can eat a variety of foods to achieve your weight loss objectives by setting these nutritional goals or guidelines. These dietary objectives are centered on your intake of protein, carbohydrates, fats, vitamins, and minerals. A more effective strategy for weight loss than counting calories is maintaining these important factors in balance with what your body requires.

STEP TWO: PLOT OUT YOUR MACROS

Not all aspects of a diet revolve around food intake. You must also make sure you are providing your body with the nutrients it requires to maintain a high level of energy, burn fat, and build muscle. The fundamental building blocks that your body uses to carry out these tasks are known as macronutrients. The majority of your daily calories come from these basic nutrients. There are three major subcategories of macros:

CARBOHYDRATES. In order to fuel muscles, simple and complex sugar chains are broken down in the body.

FATS. In order to provide emergency energy when quick-burning carbohydrates are not available, extra calories are stored in fat cells. Additionally, many hormonal and brain processes depend on fat.

PROTEINS. The body's tissues can repair and grow as a result of the material and energy that these powerful macros supply. You have the best chance of developing the body you want while not feeling deprived or worn out if you balance these macronutrients. The general recommendation is that you should consume 35% healthy fat, 40% protein, and 25% carbohydrates per day. Use an online calculator to find your ideal mix for a more customized ratio.

STEP THREE: FIND SUITABLE FOODS

Find foods that work with your new lifestyle after you've determined how much to eat. You must include foods that you'll actually eat in your diet plan if you want to lose weight. It's unlikely that you will follow your plan if you don't enjoy the food you're eating.

But it's also crucial to make an effort to explore new menu choices. Due to a restrictive diet high in empty calories, many dieters enroll in weight loss programs. The first step in developing a long-term eating strategy is to increase the number of nutritious options on your daily menu.

Find foods that work with your new lifestyle after you've determined how much to eat. You must include foods that you'll actually eat in your diet plan if you want to lose weight. It's unlikely that you will follow your plan if you don't enjoy the food you're eating.

But it's also crucial to make an effort to explore new menu choices. Due to a restrictive diet high in empty calories, many dieters enroll in weight loss programs. The first step in developing a long-term eating strategy is to increase the number of nutritious options on your daily menu.

Make a list of your favorite foods and ingredients to get started. Once you start eating healthy, try adding one or two new fruits, vegetables, or grains to your list each week. It's useful to include information on each item's macronutrient content as well because you can use this information to determine how much of each ingredient you can eat at each meal.

STEP FOUR: STOCK UP ON RECIPES

Now that you know what you can eat, start collecting a variety of recipes that feature your listed foods. Pay attention to preparation instructions. The way you cook your food has a big effect on macronutrient content.

A large recipe selection is important in your diet plan for weight loss because it keeps you from getting bored. Losing interest in daily menus is the main reason many dieters don't reach their goals. Variety ensures that you'll always look forward to your next serving. An online recipe book is a great way to store your recipes.

You can modify your recipe collection to suit your preferences if you conduct sufficient research. Are sweetbreads and pastries your favorite foods? Your favorite baked goods may be found in low-calorie varieties. Are sauces a necessary component of your daily meals? Look for homemade versions of the condiments you use the most. Do you feel anxious about giving up fried foods? Look for recipes that can simulate the crunch you crave in the oven without adding extra fat.

For those who live life on-the-go, compile a list of your most frequented restaurants. Ask the staff for nutritional information on their menu items. Use that data to create a list of selections that fit within your dietary budget.

STEP FIVE: PLAN YOUR MEAL SCHEDULE

Just as crucial as what you eat is when you eat. Our capacity to metabolize stomach contents is impacted by daily cycles that occur in our bodies. In addition, pre-existing medical conditions or variations in how your body functions can affect how you process food.

A diet plan for weight loss that adheres to the conventional paradigm of three meals per day often fails. This is particularly valid for those actively reducing their daily caloric intake. Try to separate your meals and snacks by about three hours. This prevents you from becoming overly hungry and turning to unhealthy foods to satisfy your hunger. Here are some additional suggestions to assist you in creating the ideal diet program for weight loss.

To avoid late-night snacking, eat a substantial dinner.

Eat a breakfast high in protein within an hour of waking up.

Please follow your mealtime schedule.

Consult your doctor for assistance in creating a schedule that supports maintaining the proper blood sugar levels if you have diabetes or other glucose conditions that are affected by your eating habits.

STEP SIX: TRACK, EXAMINE, AND CHANGE

To keep track of your meal plan, use a food diary. This establishes a record that enables you to review your eating patterns and assess the success of your strategy. When necessary, make adjustments to stay on course for your desired weight. If a particular diet isn't yielding the desired results, don't be afraid to switch things up. The Best Diet: The One That Works for You

The good news is that you don't need weeks' worth of pricey prepared frozen meals or a strict eating and exercise regimen to lose weight if you recoil at the thought of adhering to someone else's idea of how you should lose weight. It only takes a tiny reduction in caloric intake, ideally on a diet that meets nutritional requirements.

The author of Your Inner Skinny: Four Steps to Thin Forever, Joy Bauer, MS, RD, asserts that "one diet is not necessarily any more successful than the next." According to research studies, weight loss occurs regardless of the diet's carbohydrate composition — whether it's high in carbohydrates, low in carbohydrates, high in protein, or low in fat.

here's the catch: If you don't permanently alter your eating and exercise habits in a way that works with your schedule, lifestyle, and food preferences, your weight loss efforts won't last.

You should reflect on your own needs before creating your own diet plan.

What's Your Diet Type? knowing who you are and what you need is the most important information you can have when it comes to losing weight, eating healthfully, and changing your lifestyle."

In the book, "Use the Power of Your Personality to Find Your Best Way to Lose Weight," the author argues that "our personalities explain why some weight-control strategies succeed while others fail.

Dieting requires more than just willpower and that those who are able to lose weight and keep it off have simply found the methods that suit their individual personalities and lifestyles.

6 KEY QUESTIONS TO ANSWER

Which would you choose: three, five, or eight meals per day? Divide your calorie intake in accordance with the eating schedule you prefer.

How much time will you spend preparing food? If you don't like to cook or are short on time, you'll need to make healthy, freshly-prepared, minimally processed food preparation easier.

What kind and how much support do you need? Everyone needs encouragement to succeed, especially after the initial excitement for breaking bad habits starts to fade. You can get support from loved ones, online support groups for dieters, and diet buddies when you're tempted to give up your healthier diet and exercise routine.

Do you enjoy dining out? By looking up the calorie counts of the foods you eat the most frequently, you can account for restaurant food.

Will you need a treat every day to feel content? Reserve 100 calories for a single-serve bag of cookies or chips, or for a frozen treat like a fudge bar, if you can't go a day without a little something special.

How much physical activity is reasonable for you? On most days of the week, experts advise engaging in at least 30 minutes of moderate physical activity, like walking, but you may need to work up to that, especially if you aren't currently active. Find out from your doctor what is best for you.

CALORIE CALCULATION FOR WEIGHT LOSS

Diets are ineffective unless you create a calorie deficit by consuming fewer calories than you expend. On a balanced diet, the majority of healthy people without ongoing medical conditions shouldn't lose more than two pounds per week.

The key to any effective at-home diet plan is sticking to a daily calorie budget for weight loss. Your daily caloric intake is determined by your age, sex, level of physical activity, and weekly weight loss objectives.

Finding out what to eat to lose weight comes after calculating your calorie intake. The foundation for a lifetime of healthy eating, according to Bauer, is laid by whole foods like vegetables, fruits, whole grains, lean protein, and low-fat dairy products.

PROPOSED

Guidelines for Planning Your Daily Meals and Snacks

You are aware of the recommended serving sizes for each food category. You must now choose how to combine them to create wholesome, satiating meals and snacks that resist temptation. Here are some fundamental guidelines: Have at least three meals a day. Eating on a regular basis prevents extreme hunger that can wreak havoc on your resolve to eat better and exercise more.

Combining protein (found in foods from the milk and meat/beans food groups in the highest amounts) and fiber (found in whole grains, vegetables, fruit, and legumes) at each meal and snack will help you feel fuller for longer. Spending the same number of calories on soda crackers, which are very low in fiber and lacking in protein, is less satisfying than indulging in a snack of fat-free yogurt and an apple or a hard-boiled egg and a small whole grain roll.

Save your calories. Pick the foods from each food group that have the fewest calories. For instance, choose 93% lean ground beef instead of 85%, 1% reduced-fat milk or fat-free milk instead of full-fat, and light popcorn instead of popcorn drenched in butter.

AVOID PORTION DEVIATION BOTH AT HOME AND ABROAD

A balanced weight-control diet can include any food, but it's crucial to eat the right amounts of each. When it comes to celery and carrot sticks, most people rarely overindulge, but when it comes to cheese, pasta, fatty red meats, and other favorite foods, it's a different story.

Invest in a dependable kitchen scale, measuring cups, and measuring spoons to determine portions at home if you're unsure of what reasonable serving sizes are — and let's face it, most of us are.

When eating out, it's especially helpful to eyeball portions correctly. Since it's unlikely that you'll be eating every meal at home, having this skill is helpful.

Hope Warshaw, MS, RD, author of Eat Out, Eat Right, claims that six meals are typically consumed away from home by Americans each week.

The calories can add up even when you consume reasonable portions when you eat.

PROPOSED

According to research, restaurant food contains less fruits, vegetables, whole grains, and small fat dairy than home-cooked food and more added sugar and fat.

That really doesn't mean people who eat out frequently will always fail at dieting. Nevertheless, it is beneficial to limit eating out as much as possible by bringing food with you to work and on the go and burning off extra calories through exercise.

The calorie counts of the dishes you order can be found in books and on the websites of your favorite restaurants. Always request the items you need to keep your calorie intake in check, such as grilled meat and fish prepared without additional fat, plain vegetables, and low-fat salad dressing served on the side.

CHAPTER 5

SOLVING THE WEIGHT ISSUE

Dieting might not be the best option if your doctor advises you to lose weight because you are overweight. This is because many diets call for drastic calorie reductions or the elimination of particular foods. This strategy might be effective in the short term, but when dieters return to their old eating patterns, they typically gain the weight they lost back.

So what is the most effective way to lose extra weight? Establish a new norm and emphasize good conduct! New, healthier habits should take the place of old, unhealthy ones. Here are 5 strategies to accomplish that:

Avoid the sugary beverages. Sugary beverages with little to no nutritional value, such as soda, juice, sweet tea, and sports drinks, add extra calories. Regular consumers of sugary drinks are more likely to be overweight. Most of the time, choose water or low-fat milk.

EXERCISE. Regular exercise helps you look and feel good and can help you lose weight because it burns calories and builds muscle. Walking the family dog, riding your bike to school, and engaging in additional daily activity can all have an impact. Increase your workout intensity and incorporate some muscle-building strength exercises if you want to burn more calories.

LIMIT YOUR SCREEN TIME. Overweight people are more likely to spend a lot of time in front of screens. Establish reasonable time restrictions on your non-school-related use of the internet, video games, computers, phones, and tablets. In order to get enough sleep, turn off all screens at least an hour before going to bed.

OBSERVE SERVING SIZES. Extra calories from large portions can contribute to weight gain. Especially when eating high-calorie snacks, go for smaller portions. When dining out, consider splitting an entree or taking home half of your meal.

CONSUME FOUR SERVINGS OR MORE OF FRUITS AND VEGETABLES EACH DAY. More than just vitamins and minerals are present in fruits and vegetables. Additionally, they are high in fiber, which makes them filling. Additionally, you're less likely to overeat when you fill up on fruits and vegetables.

METHODS FOR SHEDDING POUNDS WITHOUT DIETING

Beginning of the year is a great time to concentrate on enhancing your diet and overall health. Losing weight is a big part of getting healthier for many people. Many people decide to change their diet and embark on a drastic weight loss program in January after overindulging over the holidays. However, before beginning a strict diet this year, you might want to reconsider. Even though many of these "fad diets" initially produce positive results, people frequently feel defeated by them because they are impossible to maintain over the long term without superhuman willpower, endless resources, and unlimited time! What's worse is that too rapid weight loss on a diet can lead to muscle loss. This can slow metabolism over time and eventually result in gaining even more weight back. Finally, if followed for an extended period of time, extremely restrictive diets that call for eliminating entire food groups may result in nutritional deficiencies. The good news is that you can lose weight without spending money on expensive specialty items, difficult cookbooks, or giving up your favorite foods!

For the majority of people, a realistic and secure weight loss rate is 1-2 pounds per week. Since fat stores approximately 3500 calories per pound, losing 1 lb of weight per week would require cutting 500 calories from your daily diet. To lose weight, you don't need to adhere to a strict diet. Instead of beginning a crash diet this year, try concentrating on these seven behavioral adjustments that, over time, can produce significant results. You can lose weight without feeling deprived by making the easy changes listed below, and you'll be able to keep the extra weight off permanently.

GUIDELINES FOR WEIGHT LOSS WITHOUT DIETING

AVOID DRINKING CALORIES

Drinks like soda, tea; coffee, milkshakes, and even juice are full of empty calories from sugar that cause weight gain quickly. The average 20-ounce bottle of soda has 240 calories and 12 teaspoons of sugar in it. That is more than 1.5 times the daily recommended amount of added sugar for men and more than twice the amount for one woman.

The next time you reach for a sugary drink, consider adding 12 teaspoons of sugar to your dinner instead! Alcoholic beverages are a further offender to be aware of. Despite having less sugar than soda, they are still packed with calories and could easily undo all your efforts to eat healthily. The quickest way to lose weight is to stop drinking calorie-dense beverages and switch to unsweetened or plain water.

EAT HEALTHY FOOD

You can still eat the foods you like while watching your weight. Focus on nourishing your body with foods that pack a nutritional punch, such as vegetables, fruits, whole grains, legumes, nuts and seeds, and lean proteins, rather than restricting the "bad" foods. Eat at least 1-2 cups of non-starchy vegetables first, followed by a large portion of lean proteins and nutritious carbohydrates like fruits, beans, potatoes, or whole grains. As a general guideline, split your plate in half, placing non-starchy vegetables on one half and carbs and protein on the other. You will be well on your way to a healthier diet if the majority of your meals follow this guide!

SHEDULE TREAT BEFORE TIME

When the time comes to indulge, planning what and how much you intend to eat in advance can help you avoid overindulging. Plan your treats and splurges in advance rather than trying to adhere to a Spartan diet that forbids all indulgences. You might decide, for instance, to treat yourself to a small piece of chocolate each evening or a weekly meal out at your preferred restaurant. By scheduling treats on a daily or weekly basis, you can include your favorite foods in moderation and prevent cravings, which frequently interfere with weight loss efforts.

BE AWARE OF YOUR HUNGER SIGNALS.

Ask yourself, "Am I really hungry? " the following time you reach for a treat or a snack. Frequently, we eat for reasons other than actual hunger. We eat when we are bored, worn out, emotional, or simply because there is food available. To distinguish between physical hunger and other types of needs is one of the best ways to lose weight without feeling deprived. Physical hunger symptoms can include, but are not limited to, stomach grumbling, fatigue, dizziness, or the sensation of having a "empty stomach." Recognize your unique hunger cues by yourself. If you frequently reach for food even when you're not actually hungry, consider identifying your true needs.

EAT MINDFULLY

When you eat, pay attention to your food. Make eating a time to relax, reflect, and savor each bite of food. Eating larger portions with less satisfaction can happen when eating while being distracted by work, the television, or the computer. Eat away from any distractions if at all possible. To help you eat more slowly the next time, try setting your fork down between bites or using your opposite hand. To aid in reducing mindless eating between meals, set boundaries for where and when you can eat.

Keep snacks away from your desk, for instance, and only eat in the kitchen or dining room at home.

KEEP TABS ON YOUR ROUTINES AND DEVELOPMENT

You can maintain your new habits by keeping a food journal, tracking your workouts or daily steps, and scheduling weekly weigh-ins at the same time each day. Even if you don't immediately notice any changes on the scale, you will be able to see everything you have done to lead a healthier lifestyle. If you notice that you are reverting to your old habits, keeping a food journal for a few days can help you get back on track with your weight loss goals.

A sudden change in lifestyle can be overwhelming. Choose one or two steps at a time to concentrate on for the best results. Go on to the next after you've mastered those. Remember to recognize and appreciate each healthy decision you make.

CHAPTER 6

HOW TO PERMANENTLY LOSE WEIGHT

The goal is to lose the excess weight and keep it off permanently. Unfortunately, only approximately a third of dieters are able to maintain their weight loss. Veteran dieters are aware that keeping weight off needs attention to detail, which for some people is tougher than actually losing the weight.

GETTING BETTER THROUGH PRACTICE

Something becomes simpler the more you do it. Making such good habits a routine requires time. Don't allow all your hard work goes to waste; be patient with yourself. Recognize your areas of weakness and be ready. There will be times when you'll feel tempted by particular meals or circumstances, but if your resolve is strong, you can resist temptations. The best strategy in those challenging circumstances is moderation.

One of my favorite weight-maintenance techniques is to designate a day of the week when I can indulge a little. This day must change from week to week; otherwise, you can end up having more than one "off" day per week as a result of the situation. I allow myself to treat myself to my favorite foods on my scheduled day off, which is usually a Saturday for obvious reasons. It's okay to have a small cheesecake slice, but not the entire thing! In essence, it is deliberate cheating. It works a treat for me, and it might for you as well. Even just knowing that I can relax on Saturday helps me perform well all week.

GAINFUL LOSERS

We can learn from others who have been successful in the weight-loss game. People who have dropped at least 60 pounds and kept it off for at least five years are tracked by the National Weight Control Registry (NWCR). Some of the things they do are as follows: Put it in writing. A great way to stay on track is to keep a meal journal.

Eat healthy, light food. The majority of successful losers stick to low-fat diets, as gimmicks, special diet foods, and miracle medicines are ineffective over the long haul.

DAILY EXERCISE. The favored exercise is walking, which these people schedule into their days as a must, just like cleaning their teeth.

Every day, NWCR members work out for around an hour.

START MORNING WITH BREAKFAST. The importance of getting a good start to the day is supported by all the evidence.

Regularly weigh yourself. In the event that they put on a few pounds, they instantly make changes to return to a healthy weight.

Successful losers enjoy their new lifestyles, and leading a healthy existence no longer feels like a hardship. It must be a way of life rather than just a diet. And it does grow simpler with time to maintain weight. Most likely, you're in the clear if you can make it to two years.

PROPOSED

Keep your motivation strong and don't allow obstacles derail you; if you fall off the wagon, simply pick yourself back up and carry on with your winning strategy. You can maintain your weight indefinitely if you can train your brain to think and behave like a thin person. Additionally, it gets simpler the more you practice. By the time you reach the maintenance level, it's likely that you've already discovered patterns, methods, and abilities that have helped you stay on course.

Gratify yourself. You should be commended for making positive dietary and activity adjustments that not only inspire your loved ones but also have a major positive impact on your health.

According to research, long-term weight maintenance is correlated with staying in touch with the people or programs that assisted you in losing weight. Maintaining contact with those who gave you the initial boost to success makes sense. Stay with us, and we'll help you keep the weight off.

CONCLUSSION

Regular physical activity, a reduction in saturated fat intake, a reduction in sugar intake, and an increase in fruit and vegetable consumption are all important to prevent adult obesity. Involvement from family members and medical experts may also benefit in maintaining a healthy weight.

According to a source of public health practices, there are numerous ways to influence public policy to promote measures for avoiding obesity: Possible techniques to prevent obesity include altering the eating environment, enacting policy changes in schools, and promoting medicine and other medical interventions.

There are hurdles to implementing these tactics, and just a handful of them have demonstrated to be successful.

Maintaining a healthy weight is vital for overall wellbeing. An ideal beginning step is to make an attempt to prevent obesity in your daily life. Obesity can be avoided with even minor lifestyle improvements like eating more veggies and working out a few times each week.

A dietitian or nutritionist can provide you the information you need to get started if you're interested in taking a more customized approach to your food.

Meeting with a personal trainer or fitness specialist can also assist you in identifying the physical activities that are most good for your body.

www.ingramcontent.com/pod-product-compliance
Lightning Source LLC
LaVergne TN
LVHW052059160826
845678LV00015B/3291

* 9 7 9 8 3 5 5 0 6 5 2 8 7 *